30 Days of Living Better
While Living With Pain

30 Days

of

Living Better While Living With Pain

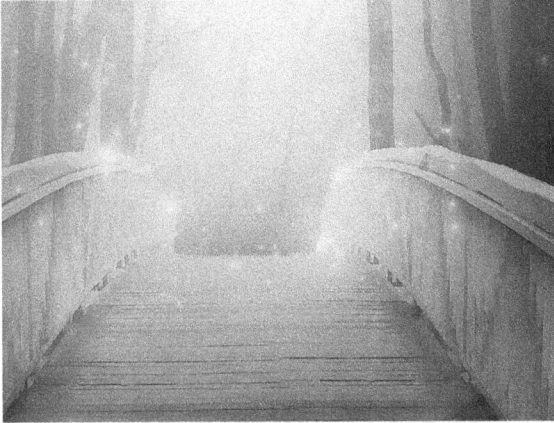

SARAH ANNE SHOCKLEY

Any Road Press

To all those who are living with pain and making the daily journey, step by step, to greater well being.

Introduction

This volume offers brief, easily digestible daily readings to help you live with more overall well being while living with pain. These are positive approaches, meditations, and suggestions that ease pain's emotional and spiritual stresses.

The daily readings are based on the principles from my popular book, *Living Better While Living With Pain.* You do not need to read that book to benefit from *30 Days*, but if you do want to read more about my approach to living with pain, the ebook version is available as a free download. It's also available in print and audio formats, if those are preferable.

I wish you all the best on your journey to healing. I always remind myself and others that life with pain is like a landscape, or a terrain, that we're traveling through. It is not the totality of who we are.

May these words and images help you navigate your personal path through pain's inner landscape and beyond it to the other side.

30 Days

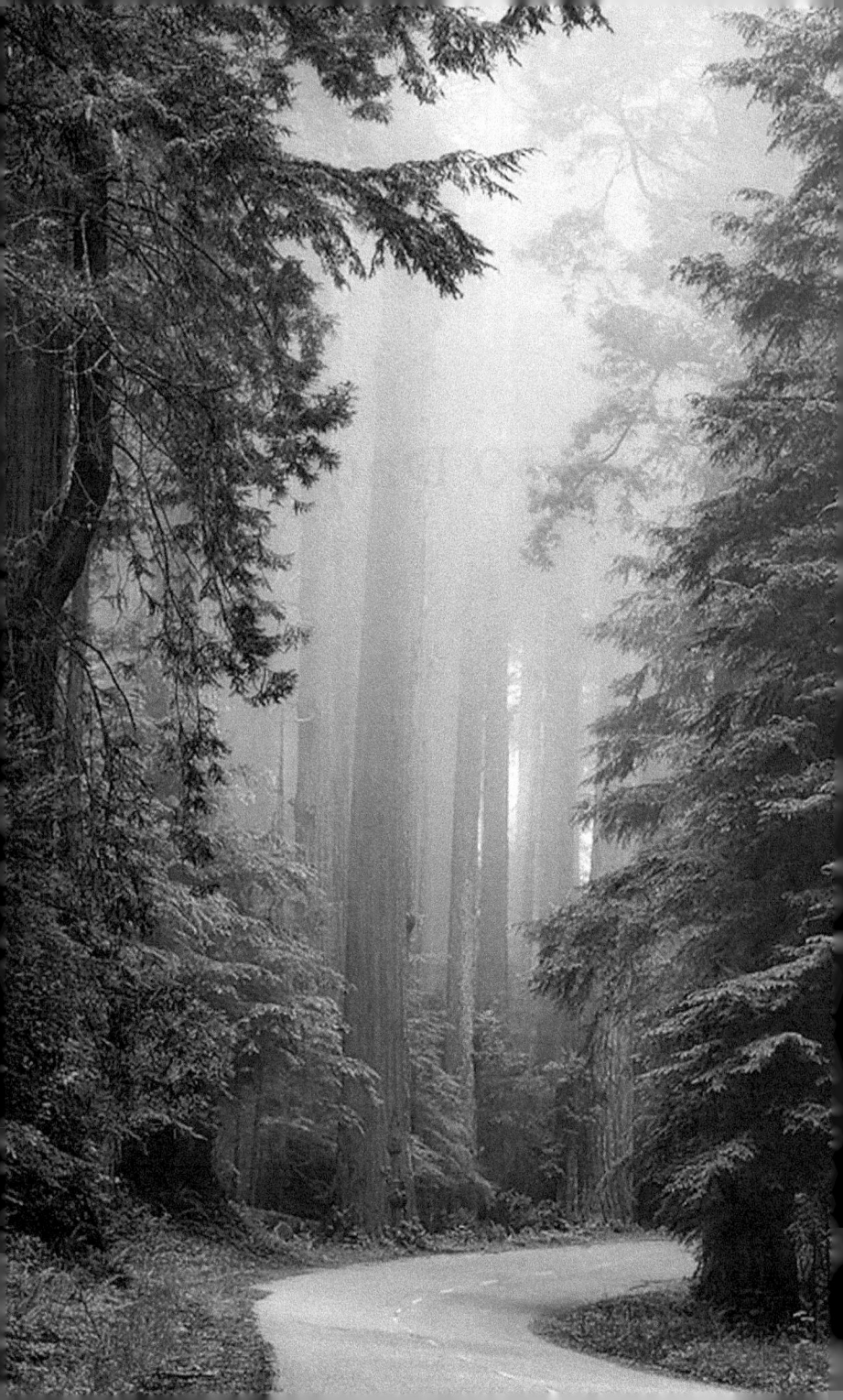

The Road

Today, I am one day closer to healing than I was yesterday.

In ways I may not understand yet, I am a day wiser, a day further down the road, a day nearer to whatever it takes to get to the other side of this pain.

I affirm this today.

I congratulate myself for taking the next step, no matter how small or how tentative; for finding ways to trust life; for finding new ways to express myself, and for finding ways to trust the path I'm on, even in this pain.

2

One Good Thing

Today, I find one good thing I can hold close to my heart and love, despite the pain.

I find one thing that is outside of this pain bubble I live in, that is still there for me, unscathed and untouched.

A flower.

A smile from a friend.

A child's drawing.

A poem.

A beautiful piece of art.

The sunset.

The moon.

The night sky.

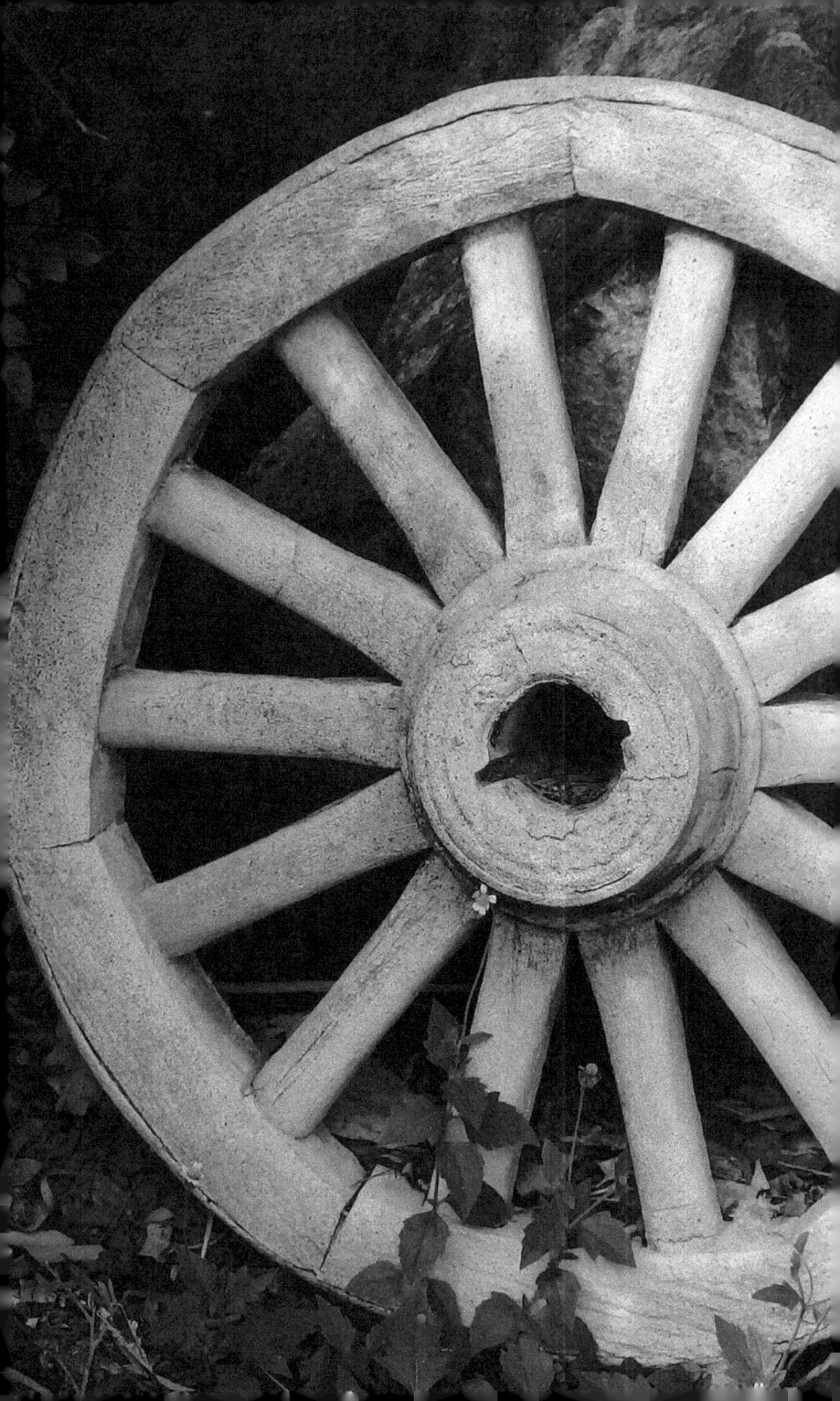

3

The Turning of the Wheel

I am part of the great wheel of life.

I don't understand why I'm here in this pain.

But I do know that as long as I am on the wheel of life, as it keeps turning and turning, my life turns with it, from dark into light, from pain into release.

I notice what has already turned for the better, and if something has turned for the worse, I remind myself that this is not the end of the story. The wheel is still turning.

The wheel turns from dark to light, from light to dark, but each turn into the dark does not have to be as dense or as heavy, as the last.

I am on a journey. This pain is part of it. This wheel, this turning, is part of it.

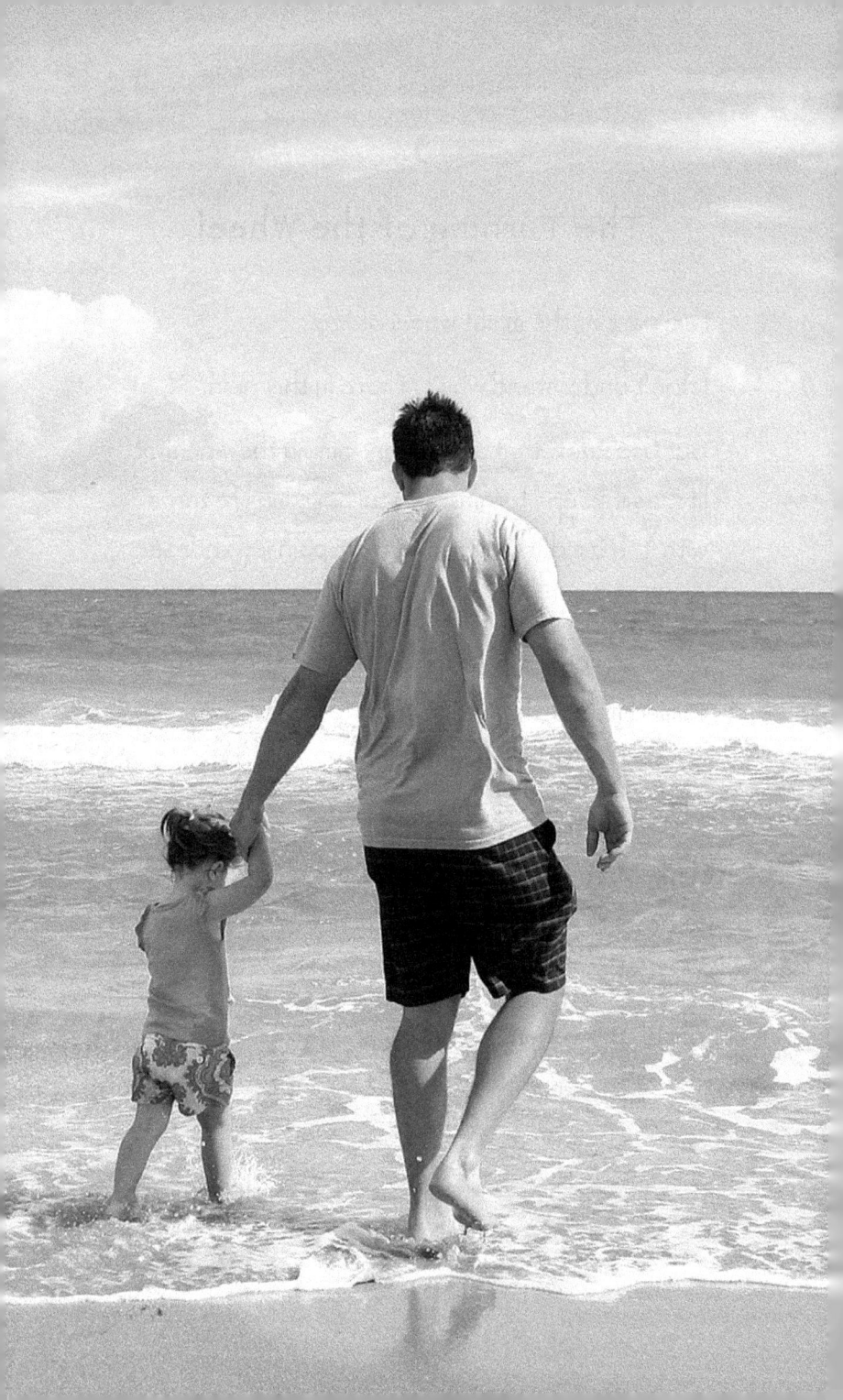

4

Reclaiming Life

Today, I reclaim the art of enjoying my life.

I have given pain a lot of room in my life. In a way, I moved over for it.

Perhaps pain will not readily move over for me, and I understand that. It is the nature of pain.

So, today I do one thing I love to do, even if it's only for a brief time, and even if pain has to come with me.

I would rather share the experience with pain, if I must, than not have it at all.

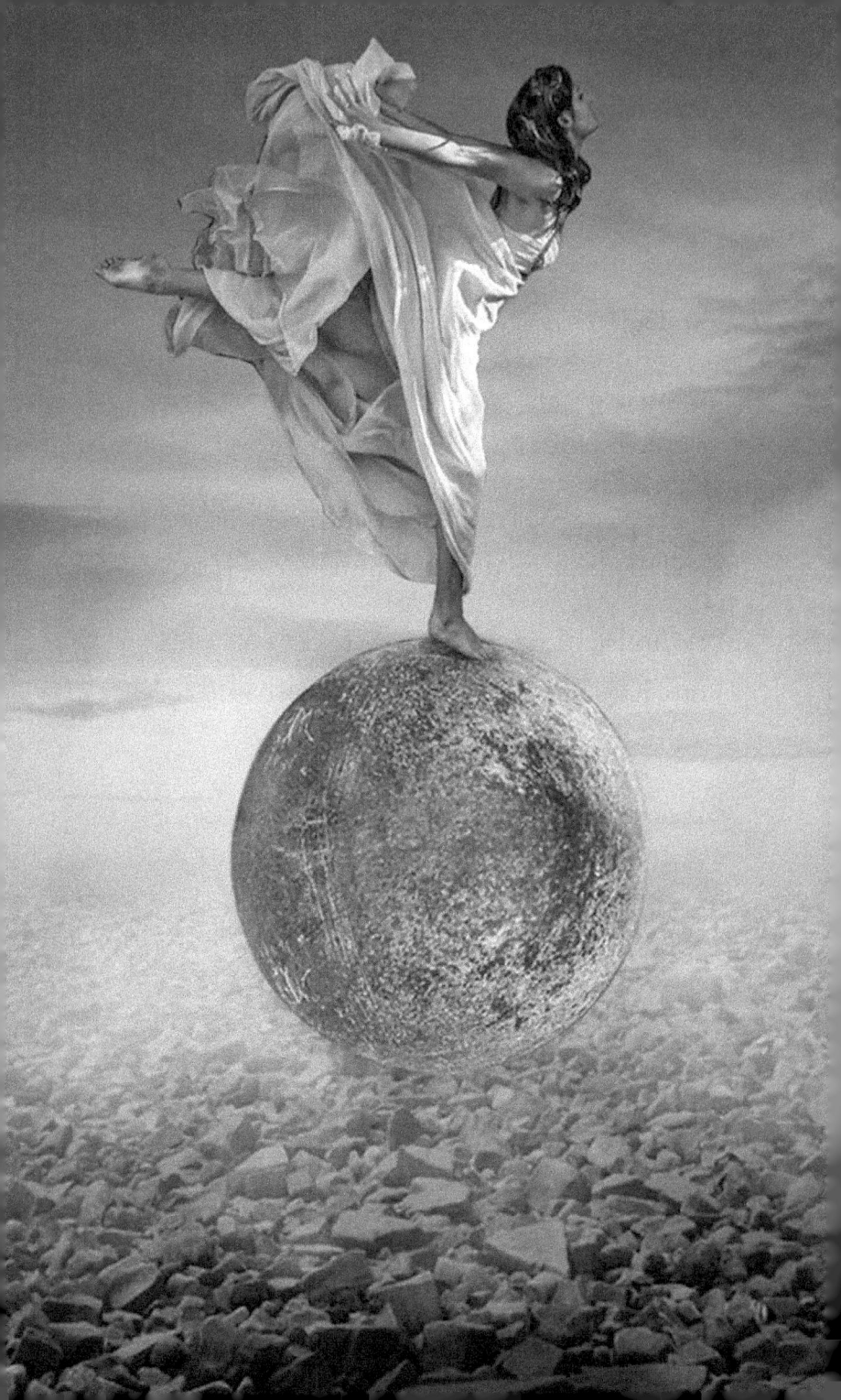

5

Remembering How to Dream

Today, I remember how to dream.

What would I prefer to be doing if I could push a button and stop the pain? Where would I most want to be and with whom?

Today I do something that shows I believe in my dreams of the future. It may be only a small gesture, a purely symbolic act, but it is a beginning.

This gesture says: I will get through this. I will survive, I will endure, I will grow, and I will dream my way into a life that includes more and more of who I want to be, even as I move through pain to get there.

6

Eyes to the East

The way is dark and I feel lost. How do I know if I'm headed in the right direction?

If I keep following the path of what feels best to me, what feels right, I will get there. If I keep my face to the East, the sun will eventually rise.

How do I keep my face to the East? I continually raise my eyes up. I keep looking toward the horizon. I keep following what feels best for this day.

Today, I notice which direction my East lies in by finding what inspires me, what makes me feel even a tiny bit more relaxed, and what feels like a lightening of the load, however slight.

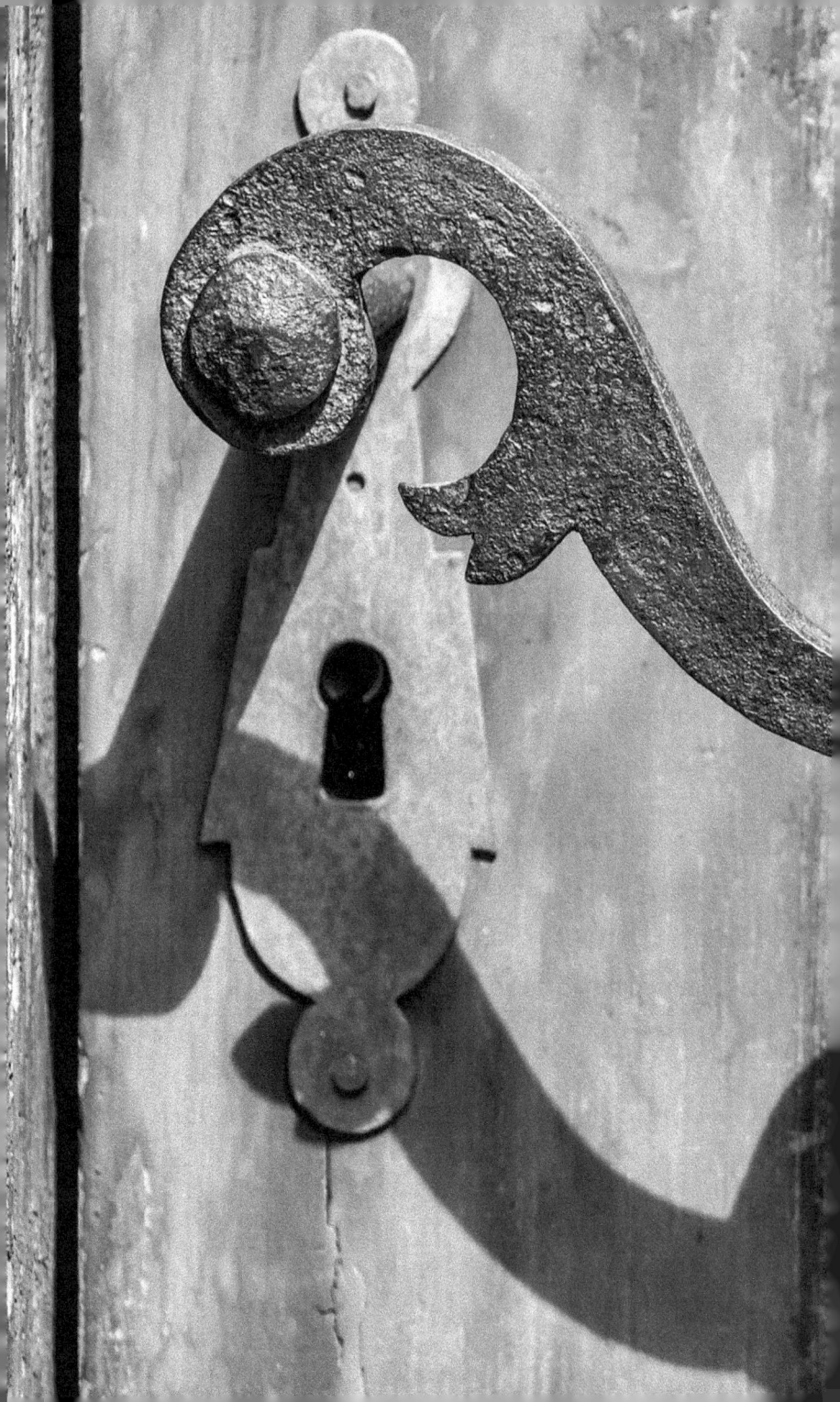

7

The Door Inside

There is a door inside of me I cannot see, but I know it is there.

Somehow, this pain points to that door. Maybe pain *is* the door.

I can open the door now or later. I can pull it open only a crack, or I can walk right through to see what is there beyond the pain.

In my imagination I reach out inside myself, take a deep breath, and turn the handle.

I find a way to express what I sense beyond that door. I write about it, or I make a drawing or collage, or I sing, or dance, or act it out.

Today, somehow, some way, I connect with what lies beyond the door of pain within my secret self.

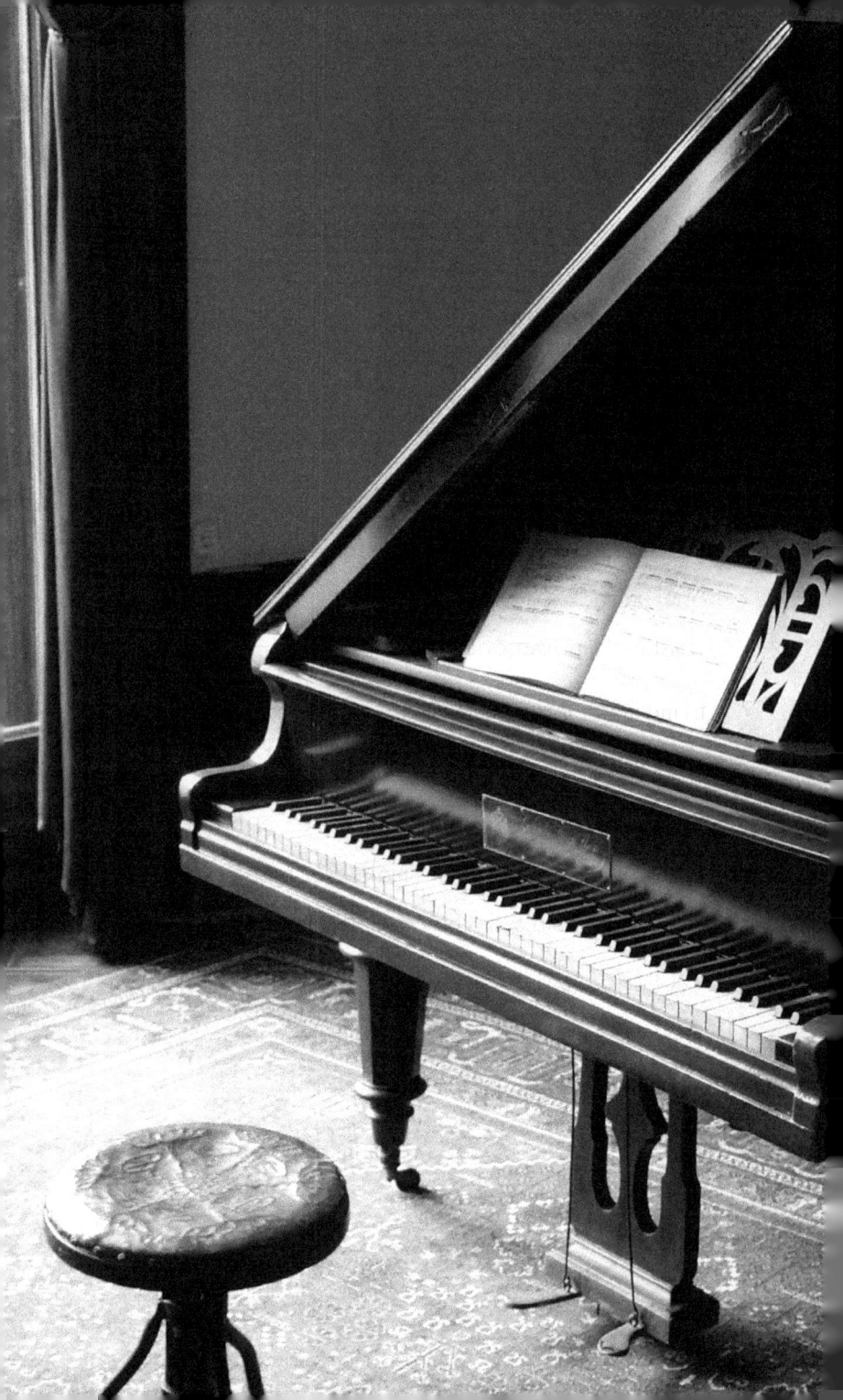

8

Sounds That Heal

Today, I listen to sounds that soothe my nerves.

I sit or lie and listen to classical or ambient music, or light guitar, flute, or piano.

I might listen to a recording of the rain or the wind or the ocean waves.

I let the sounds enter my body and move through it gently, like a caress. I let the sounds pour over my body and soothe it softly. I listen to these sounds, this music, with my whole body.

I invite my pain to listen too.

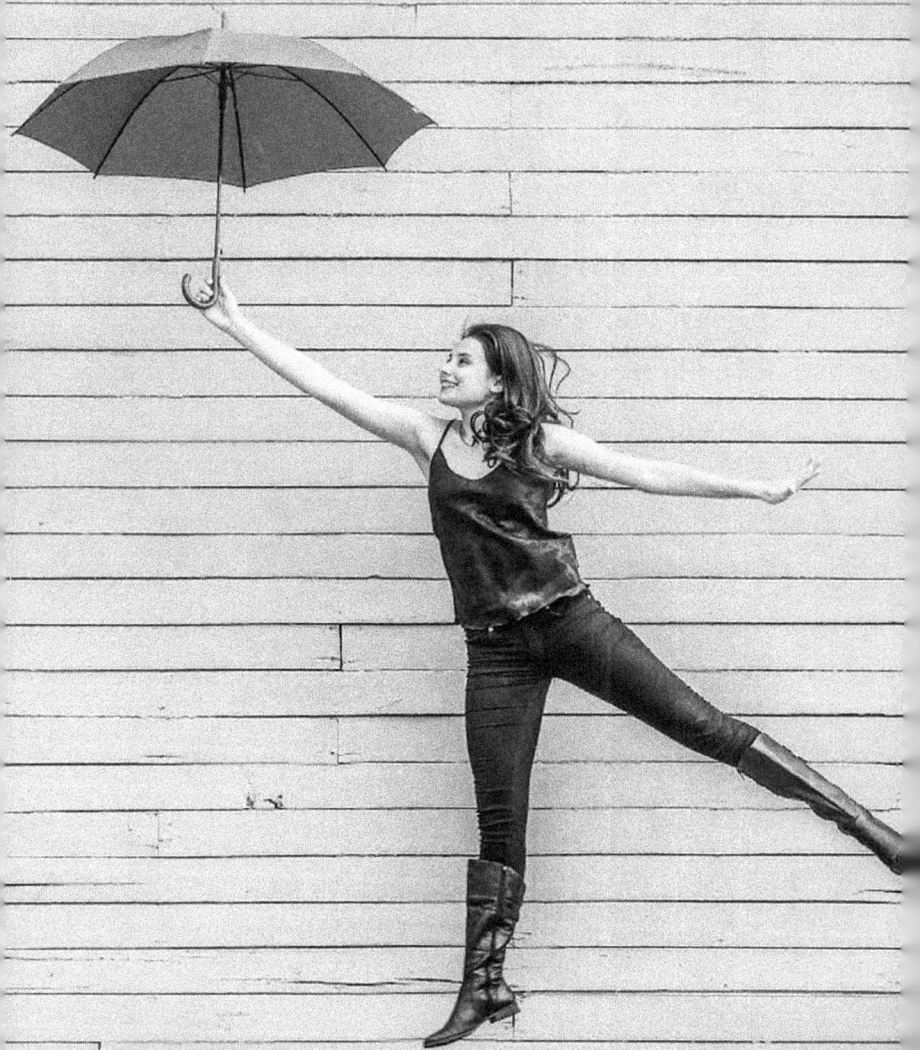

9

Laughter

Today I reclaim something valuable I thought I had lost to pain, something no one can live well without.

Today, I find at least one reason to laugh.

And then another, if I can.

And another.

Today, I reclaim my humor, and my ability to be lighthearted, even if it's just for the duration of a silly movie.

Because if I can laugh once, even in this pain, I can laugh again.

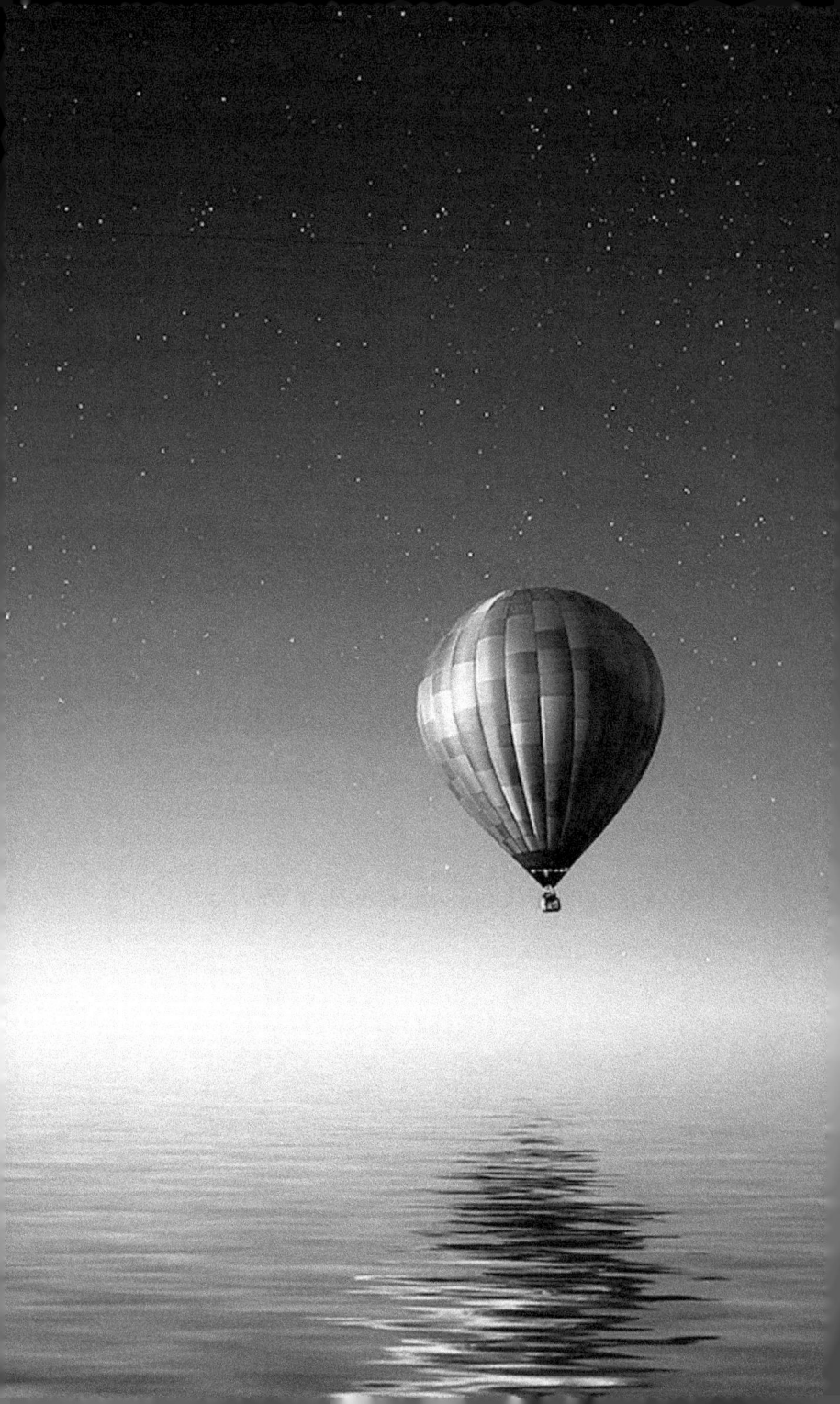

10

Freedom

Just for today, I stop arguing with life about my situation.

I stop fighting with the pain I am in.

I stop fighting myself.

I take a deep breath and ask: What would I like instead?

Then I give myself the closest thing to it that I can find or create.

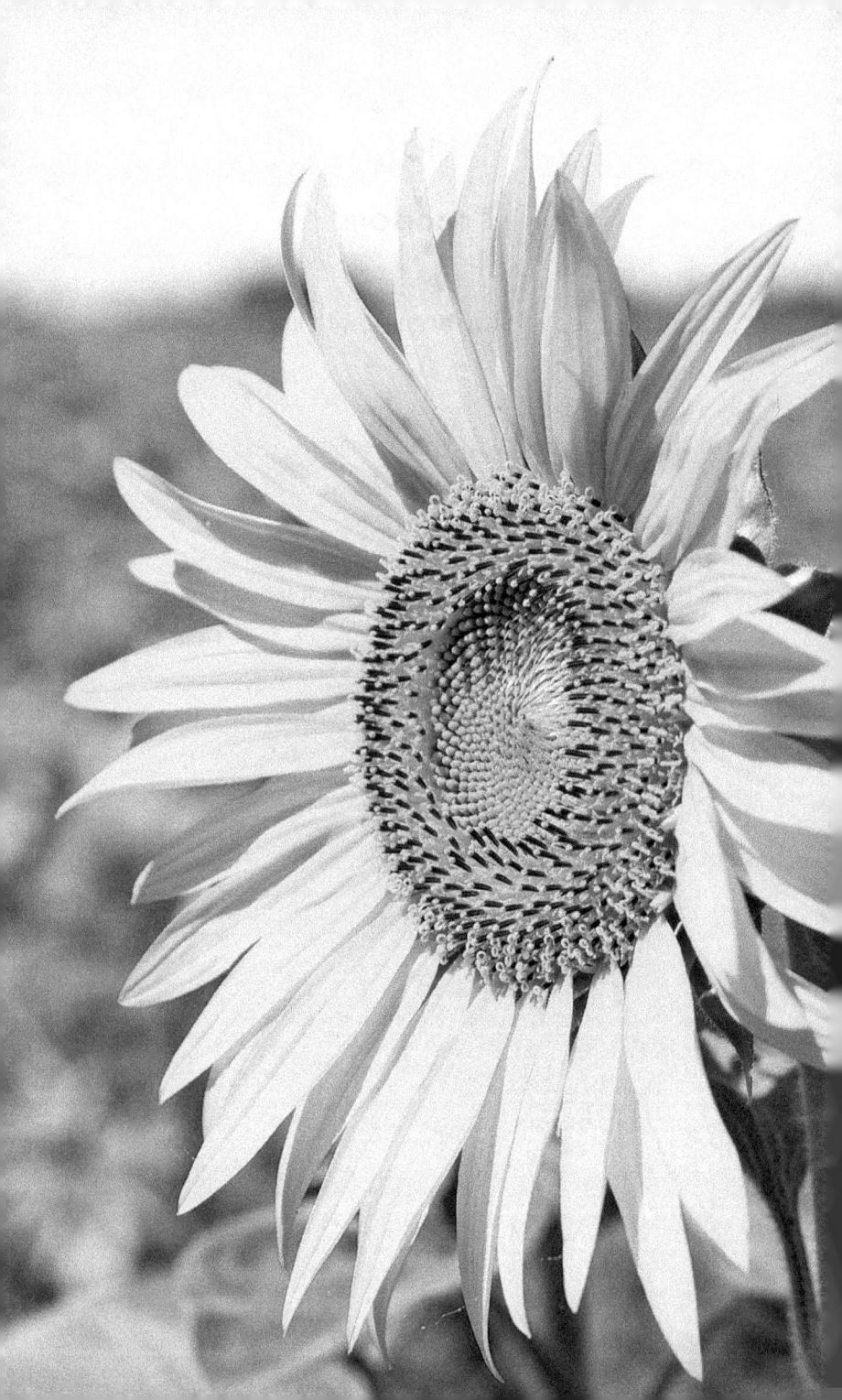

11

Breaking the Sameness

I have been in this pain long enough to feel the sameness of it, the patterns that repeat themselves, the sense of futility and loss.

Today, I choose to make a change in all that.

Today I choose to learn something new.

A foreign language. A memorized poem. The recipe for something delicious. Anything that interests me. And tomorrow I will continue.

Learning does something for me. It exercises my brain that sometimes seems to atrophy while I'm in pain. It gives me a sense of forward movement where there may have been very little before. It renews my sense of having a future because I can see progress and I can create a goal to work toward.

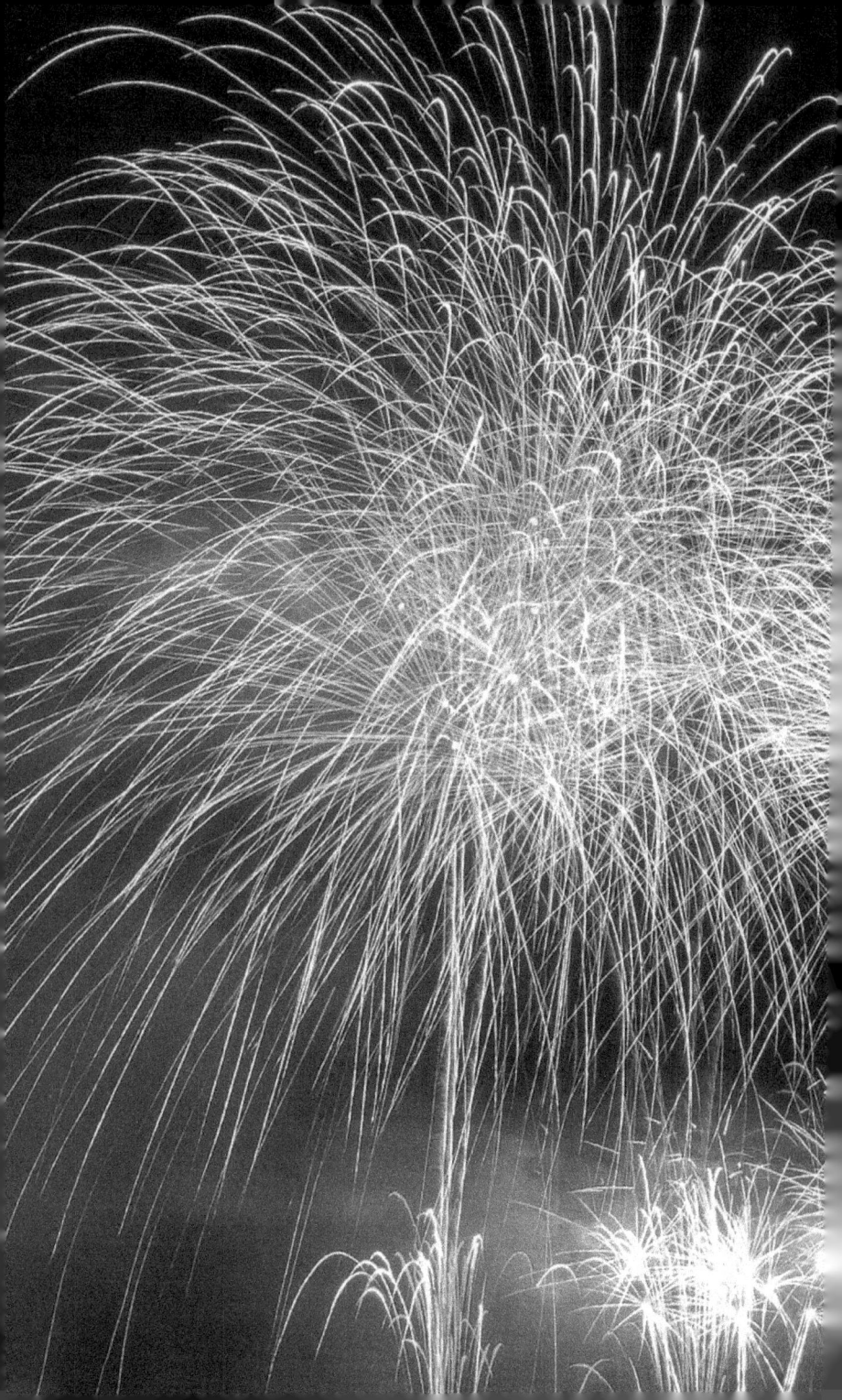

12

Renewal

What will I do the minute this pain ends?

Today, I indulge myself in imagining that moment.

In my mind, I spend some time in the hours and days right after the end of this pain.

I let myself revel in it, relax into it, feel the joy, the relief, and the sense of renewed inspiration.

What can I do that's most like that moment right now?

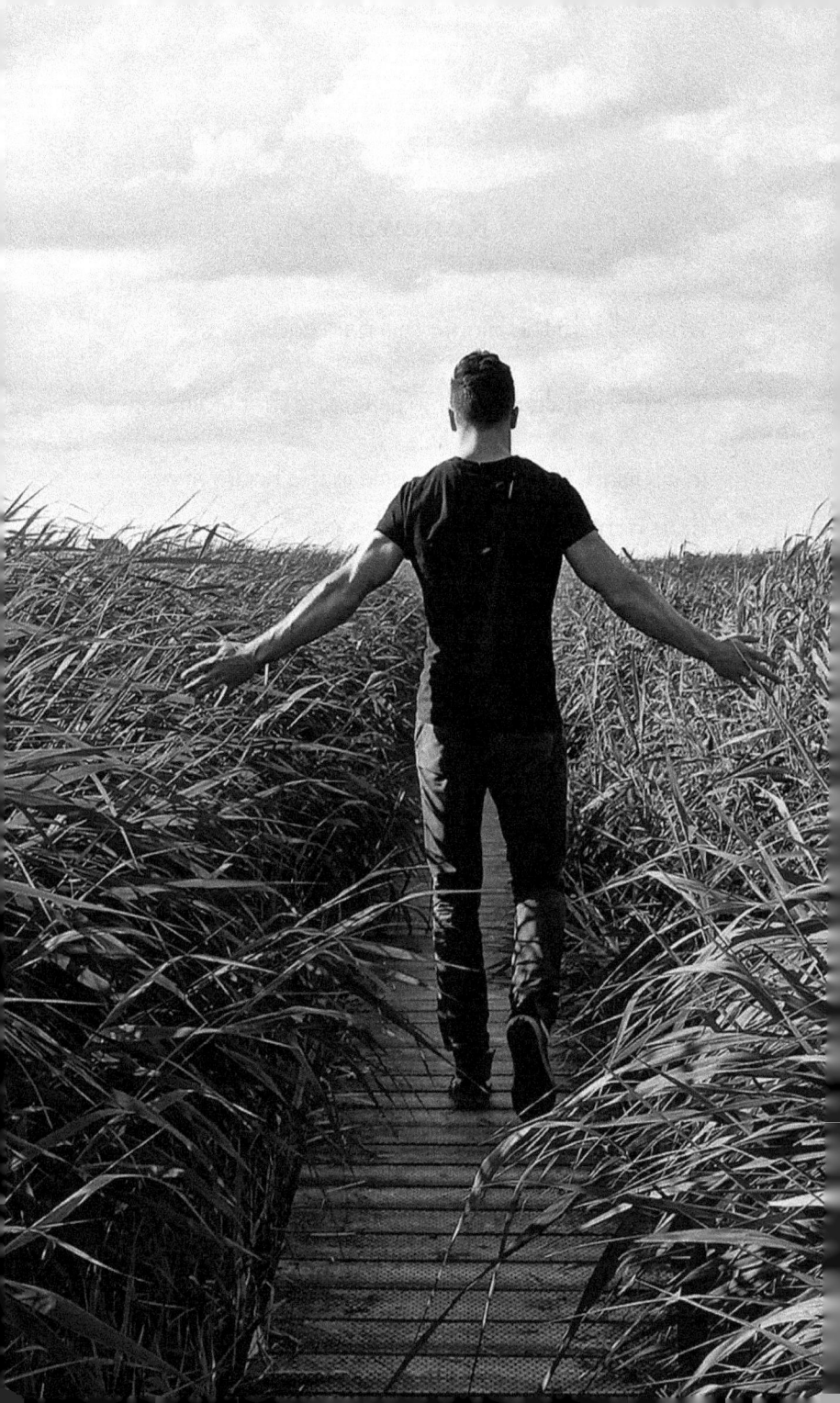

13

The Outing

Today, I take my pain on an outing, even if it's only in my mind.

Of course, I can't go anywhere completely without pain, but I can be with it differently.

Pain, I say breezily, would you like to go for a walk? A drive? A bike ride? Have a spot of tea at a nice café? Visit the library? Go to a movie? The beach? The woods? See a friend?

Today, instead of hating this reality, instead of pushing against what is true, today I *choose* to invite pain along.

And then I notice how different that is.

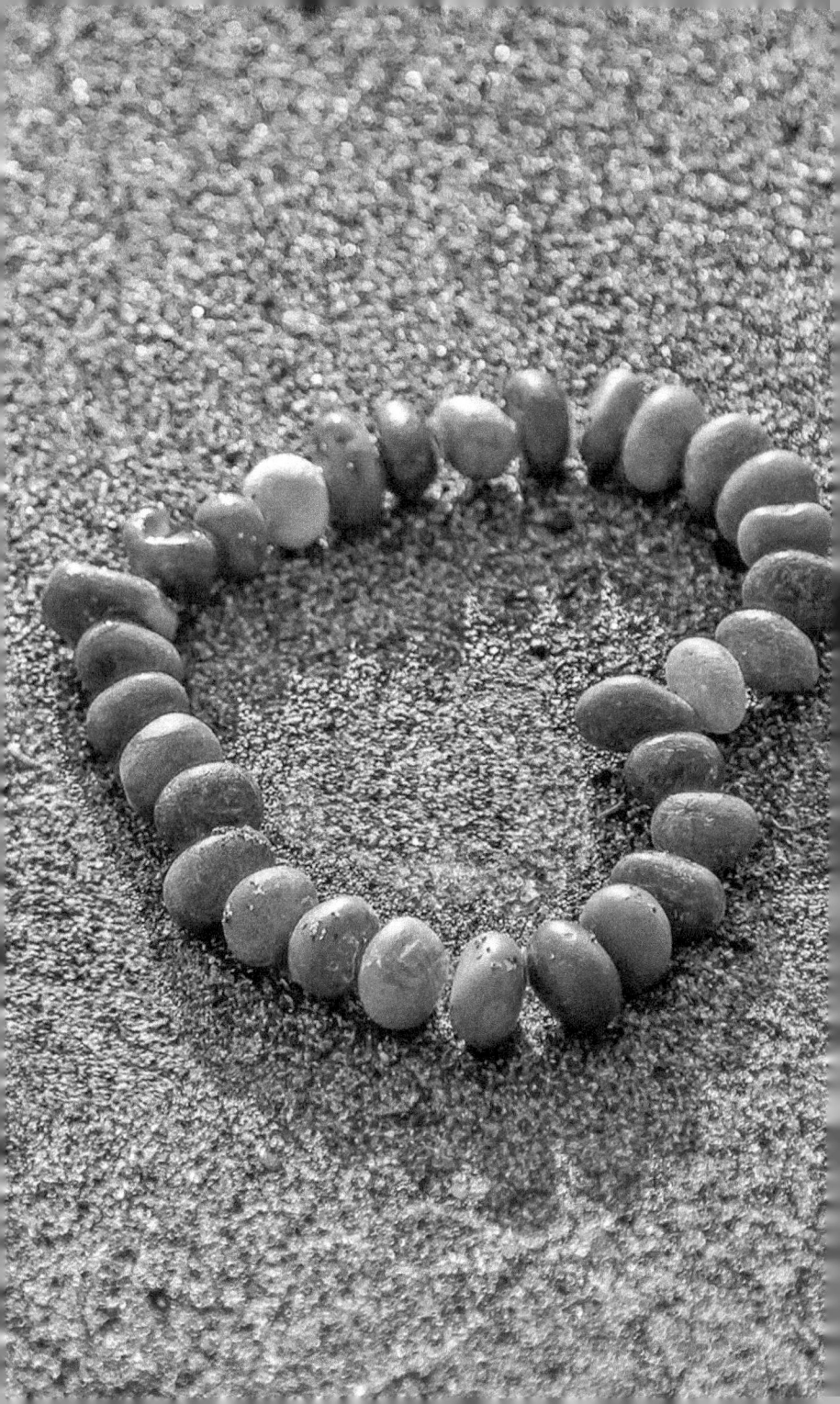

14

Connection

Pain makes me necessarily pay a lot of attention to my own needs. I may forget to connect with others because I don't always feel up to it, or I don't want to be a burden.

In this land of pain, because I feel so lacking, so compromised, and so isolated, I can easily forget that I have a presence and a comfort to offer others.

Today I will connect with someone who is experiencing loss or hardship and be the best friend I can be.

And in the process of offering my presence to others, I find I am more present to myself.

15

Pain Is Not Me

Today, I make a point to appreciate the people and the places in my life that I care about.

This pain is not my whole life, and it is not the whole of me.

I can also pay attention to other things like the beautiful day, my friendships, and my family.

I can feel this pain and still live and love and appreciate myself and others.

They are still there for me, even when my capacity for participating is diminished for the moment. I can still be thankful for what they mean to me, and I can let them draw at least part of my attention away from the pain for a time.

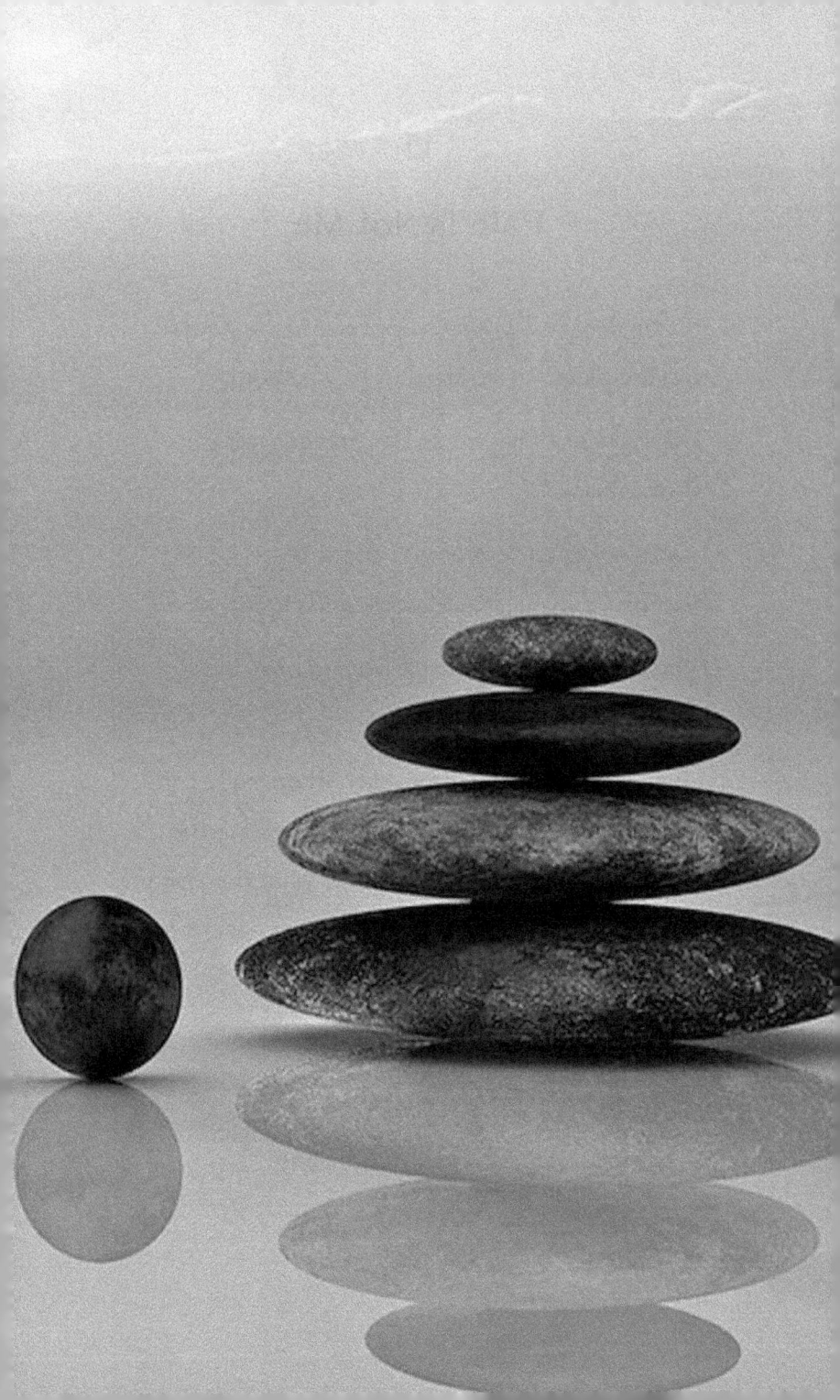

16

Balance

Have I asked anyone for help lately? Did I forget? Am I reluctant to ask for anything at all?

Or did I slide to the other end of the scale and wear everyone out?

Today I will be mindful of how much I ask of others and how often I don't ask when it would serve me better to let others help.

Today, I will try to be in balance with my own needs and the needs of others. I will remember that it is alright to take what others offer, and I will be mindful of both my limits and their limits.

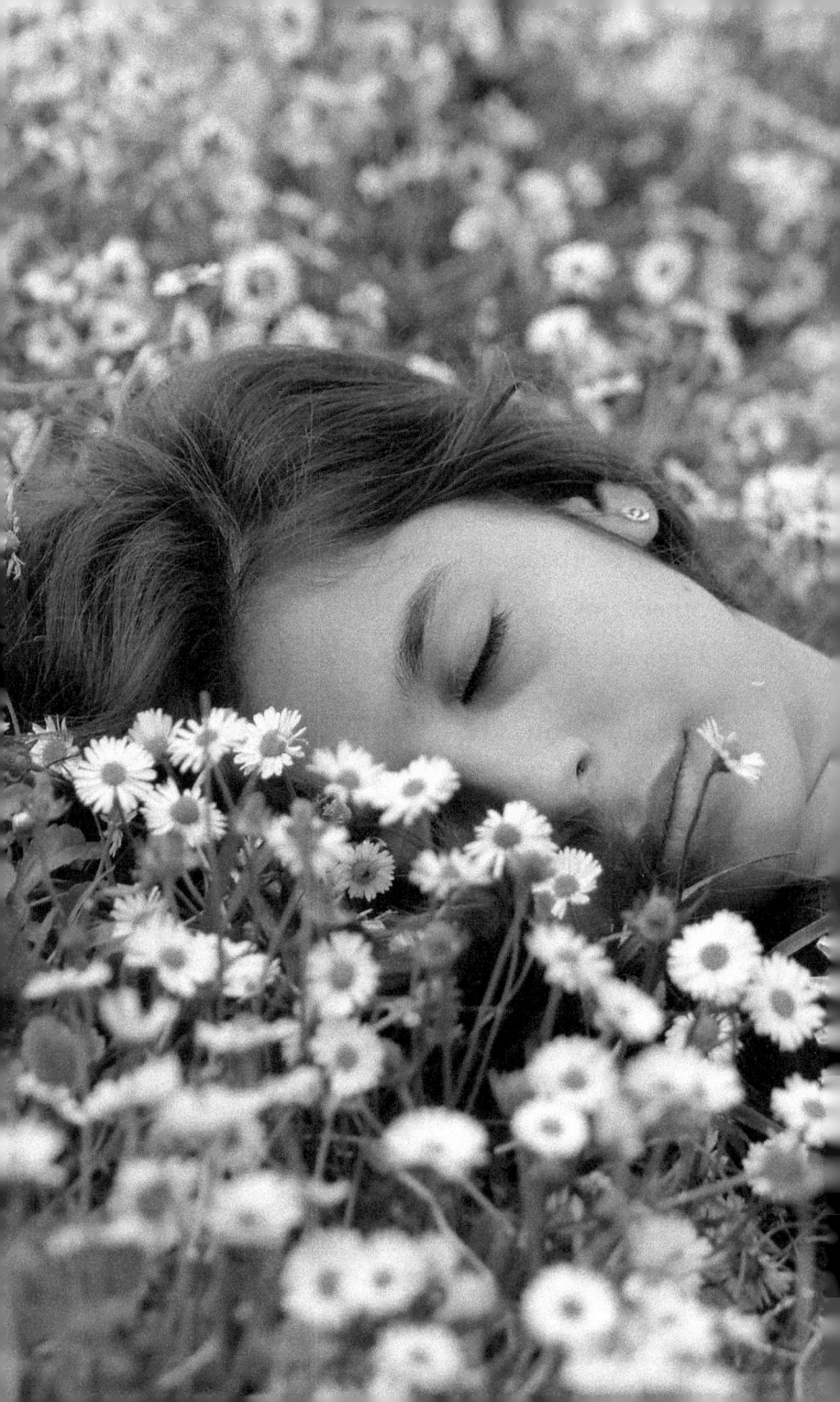

17

Finding The No-Pain Places

Today, I decide to pay special attention to those body parts that aren't in pain.

I say: Pain, I know you're still here and I know you'll be here when I get back, but just for a moment, I'm going to put most of my attention on part of me that doesn't feel you.

I'm going to feel how right and good and not in pain that part is. Just for a moment. Then, I'm going to take a little tour of my body, finding other spots of real estate that aren't in pain.

I marvel at the fact that I can actually recognize and feel the no-pain of my pinky or my toe or my ear even while you, pain, are still here in another part of my body. It's a mini-vacation.

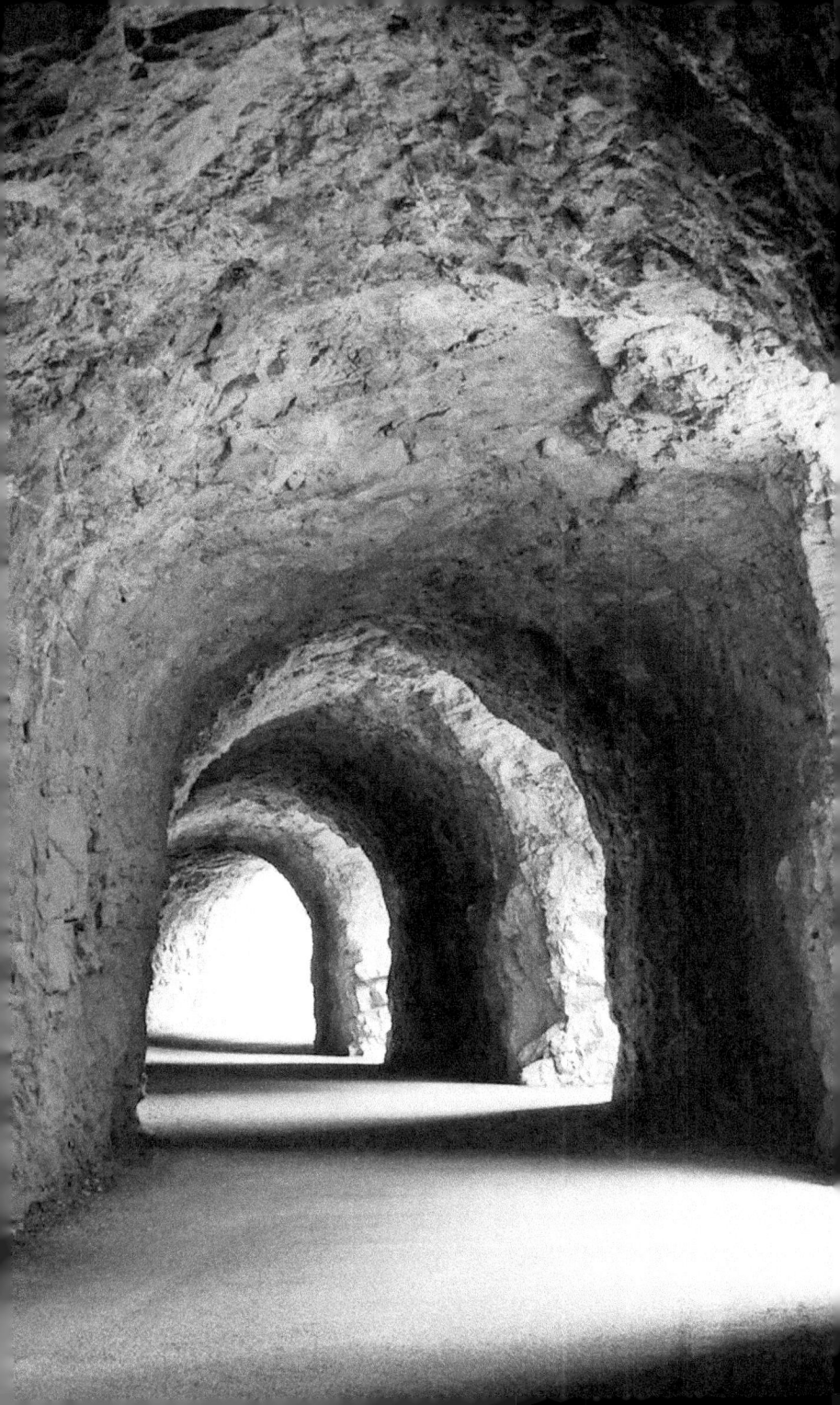

18

The Glimmer

If there's a way in, there's a way out.

I got into this pain, and I can find my way through and out.

Today, I consciously look for the light at the end of the tunnel – even if it's only a tiny glimmer.

As long as I can see a glimmer I can walk toward it.

If I can't see the glimmer yet, it might mean I have my eyes squeezed shut, or it might mean that I have to walk on just a bit further.

Because there is always a light at the end of the tunnel, no matter how dark it appears, and no matter how long the journey seems to be.

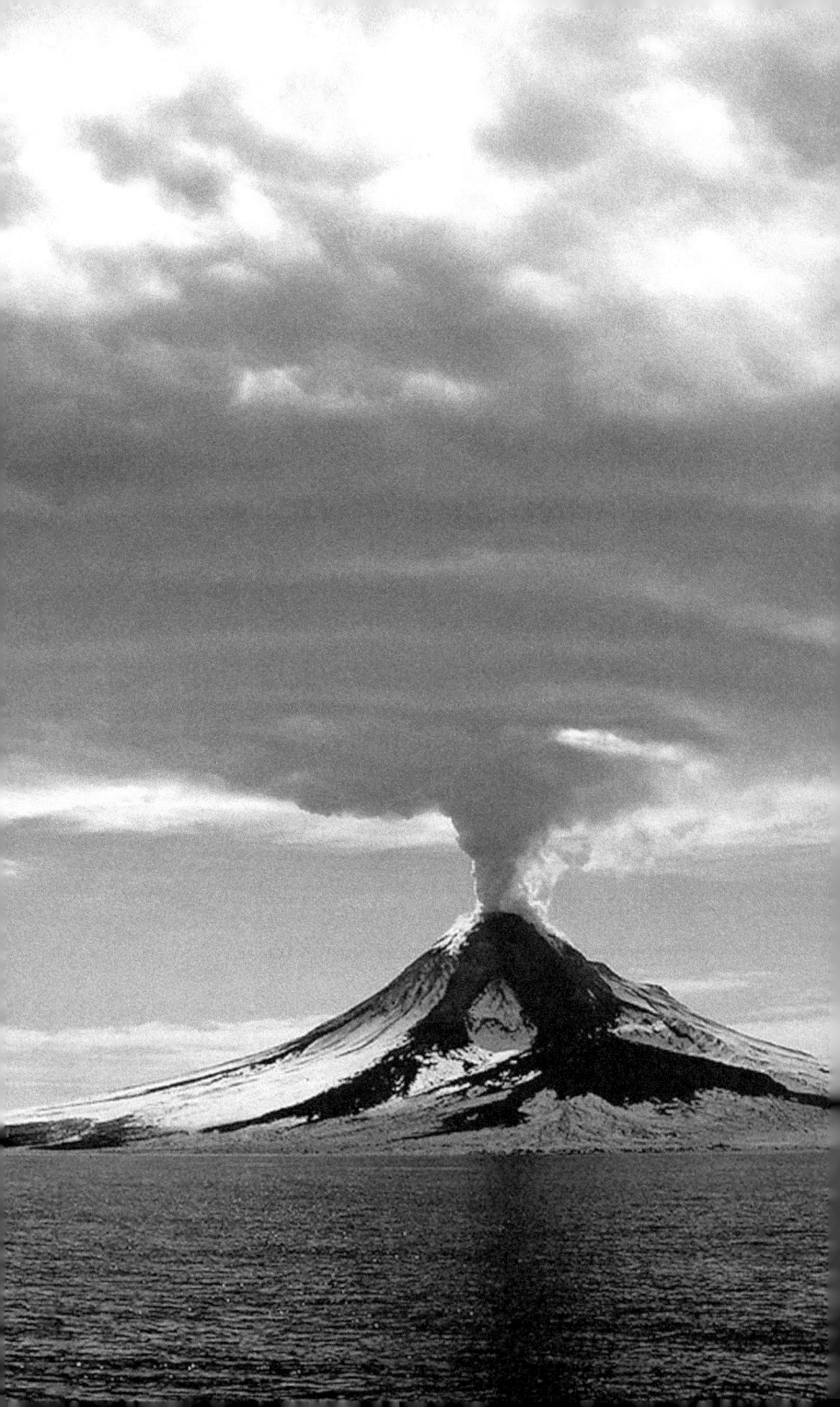

19

The Rant

Today, I give myself ten full minutes to rant and rage about this pain, this condition, this situation.

Shouted, whispered, written, or howled. I let it out.

In the shower, into my pillow, typed into my computer, or in my car.

Ten full minutes.

And then I breathe.

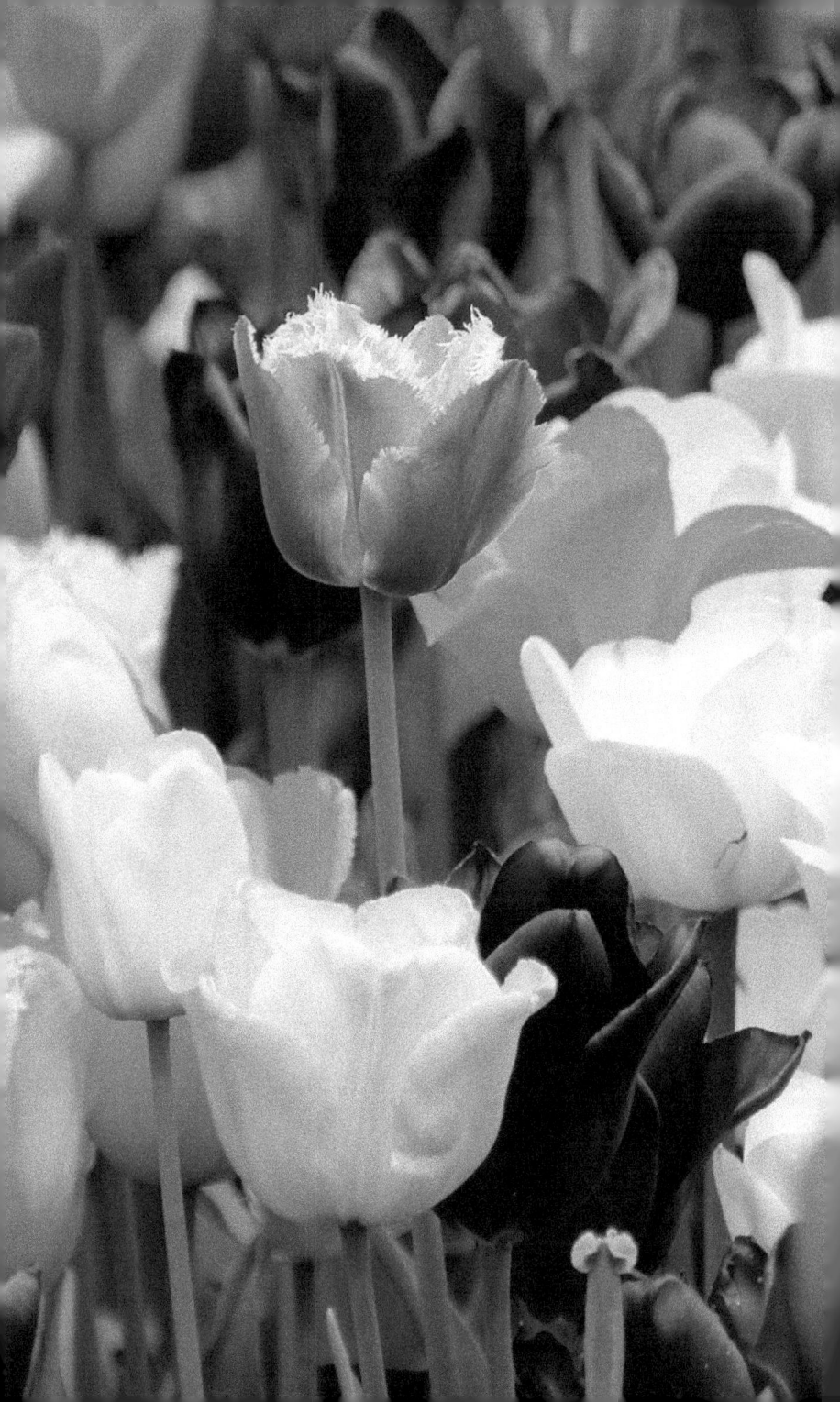

20

Life Beyond Pain

Today, I find something unusually nice to do for myself that does not involve taking care of pain.

Today, I reconnect with the self that I am without this pain—the me that dreams, the me that loves freely, the me that expresses fluidly, the me that loves who I am.

Today, I give myself the gift of something special, something fun, something beautiful, something sentimental, something wild, something soothing, or something daring that caters to the me that lives in the pain free zone.

Because, no matter how much pain most of me is experiencing, there is always a part of me that lives beyond it.

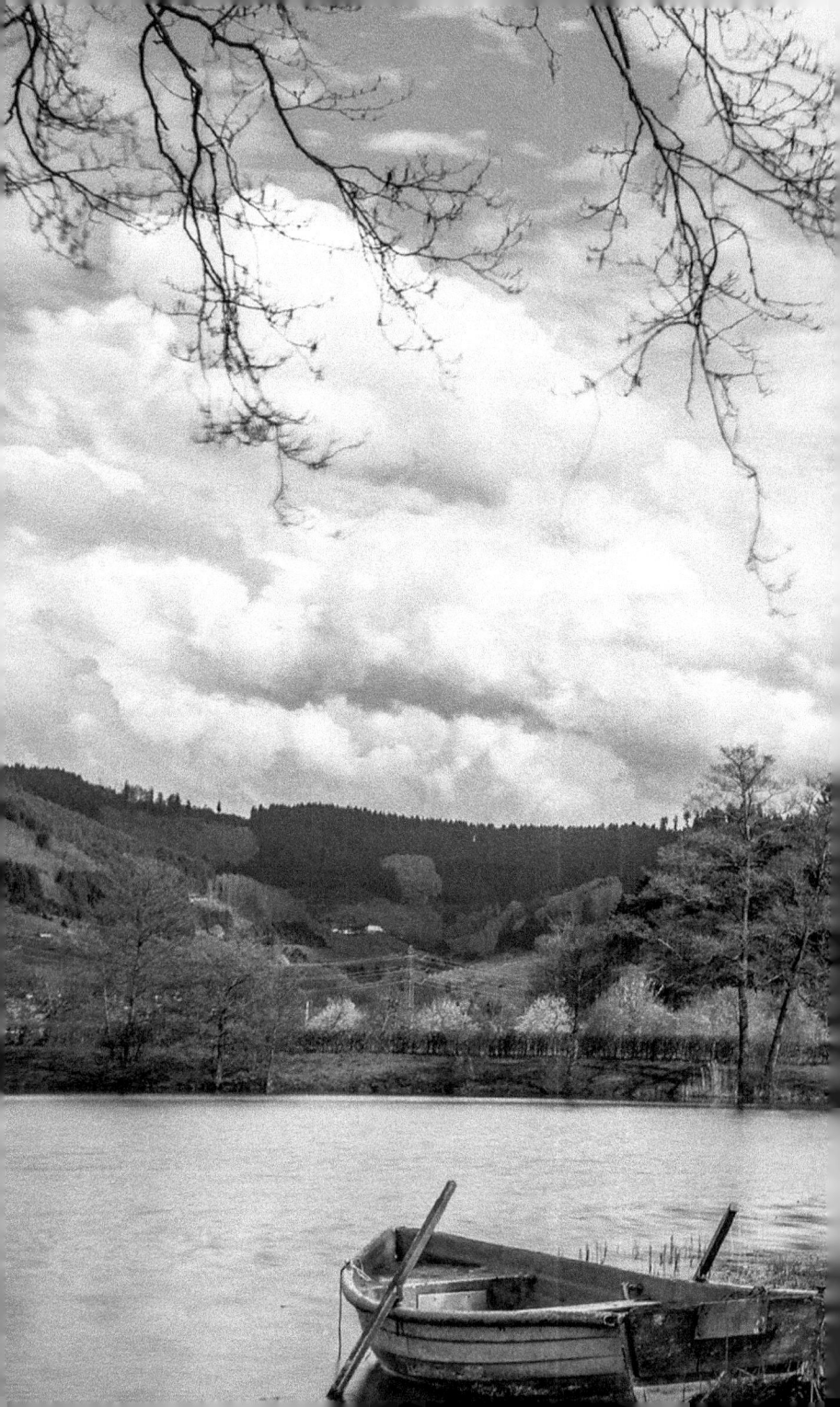

21

Peace of Mind

Today, I take a break from worry. I may have a lot on my mind, but if there's nothing I can do about things right now, I'm going to put my worries and concerns away for a day.

I imagine putting them into a box or a drawer or a storage chest. I know they will be safe there until tomorrow.

Then I give myself the gift of relaxing into greater well being. For this day, I let my body have the benefit of healthful peace of mind, relaxation, and greater well being.

The more often I can do this, the more positive effects it will have on my health, and the less acute pain I'll be in. And that will give me less to worry about.

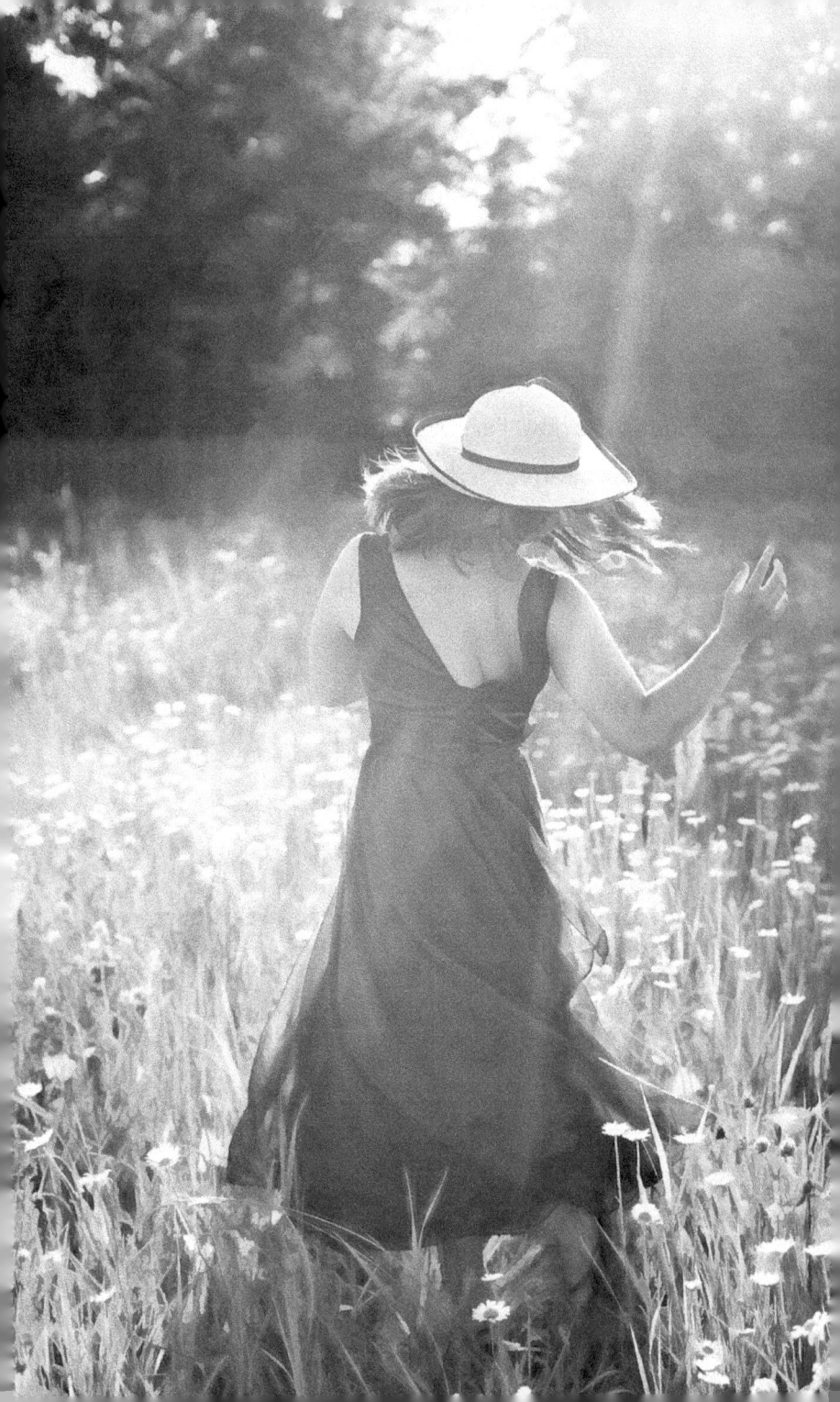

22

Returning to Life

It's easy to forget what life was like before this pain, as if pain has always been here, and always will be.

But that's not the truth. This pain has not been here all my life. There was a beginning. And since there was a beginning, I can imagine an end.

Today, to remind myself that there is life outside of this pain, I find one thing I used to love doing before the pain came and I find a way to do it, even a little, and even if it's in my imagination.

And tomorrow, I do it again. And every day that I am able. I remind myself of who I was. Who I really am. Who I want to be.

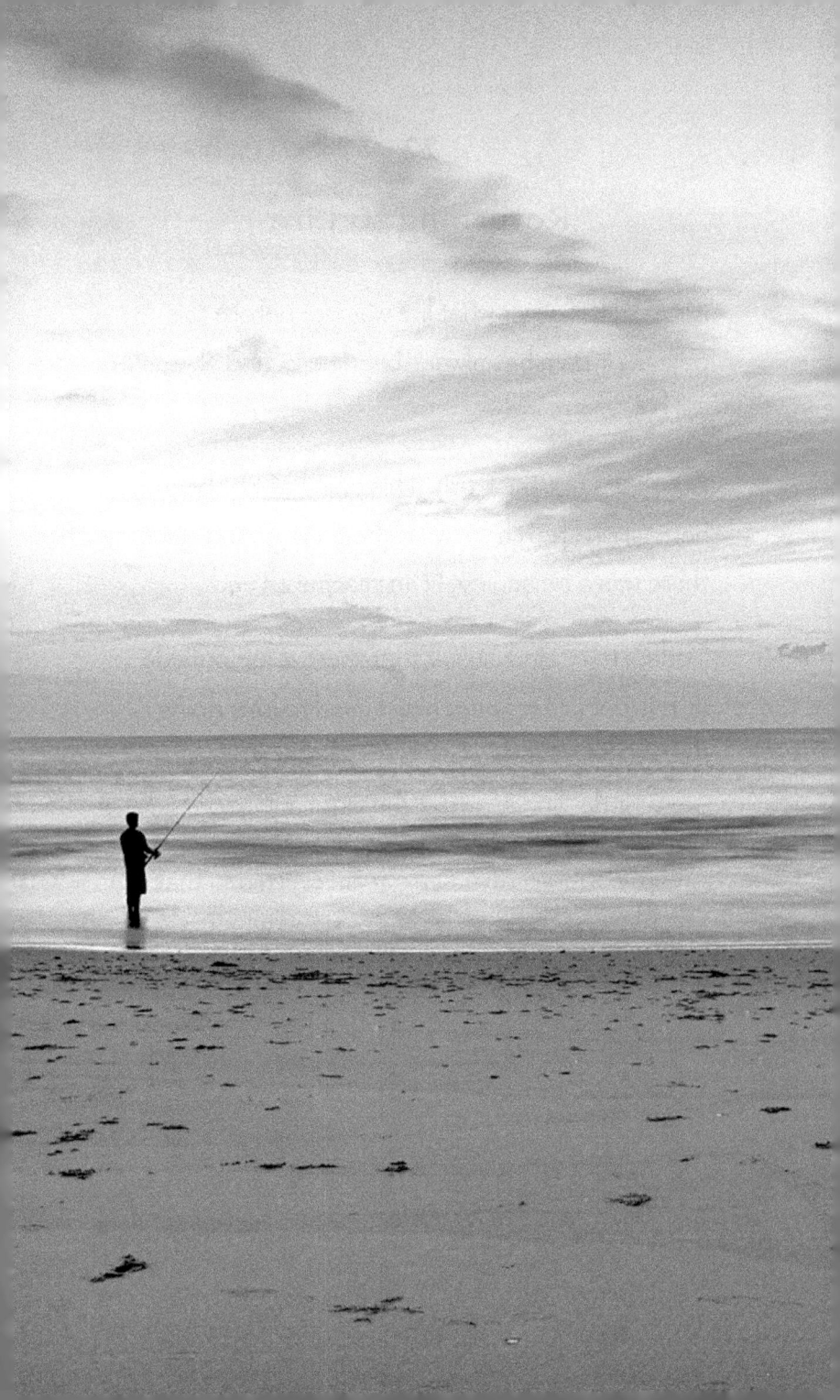

23

Lines Into The World

Being in pain can be very lonely, so today I throw lines of connection out into the world.

I attend a meeting, call a friend, go to church, find a meet-up group or participate in an online chat.

Each one of these is a line connecting me with the world. They help tether me to Life when I feel submerged by pain.

Sometimes all I can do is think about them, these lines, but just knowing they're there, that I've cast them out, helps keep me afloat.

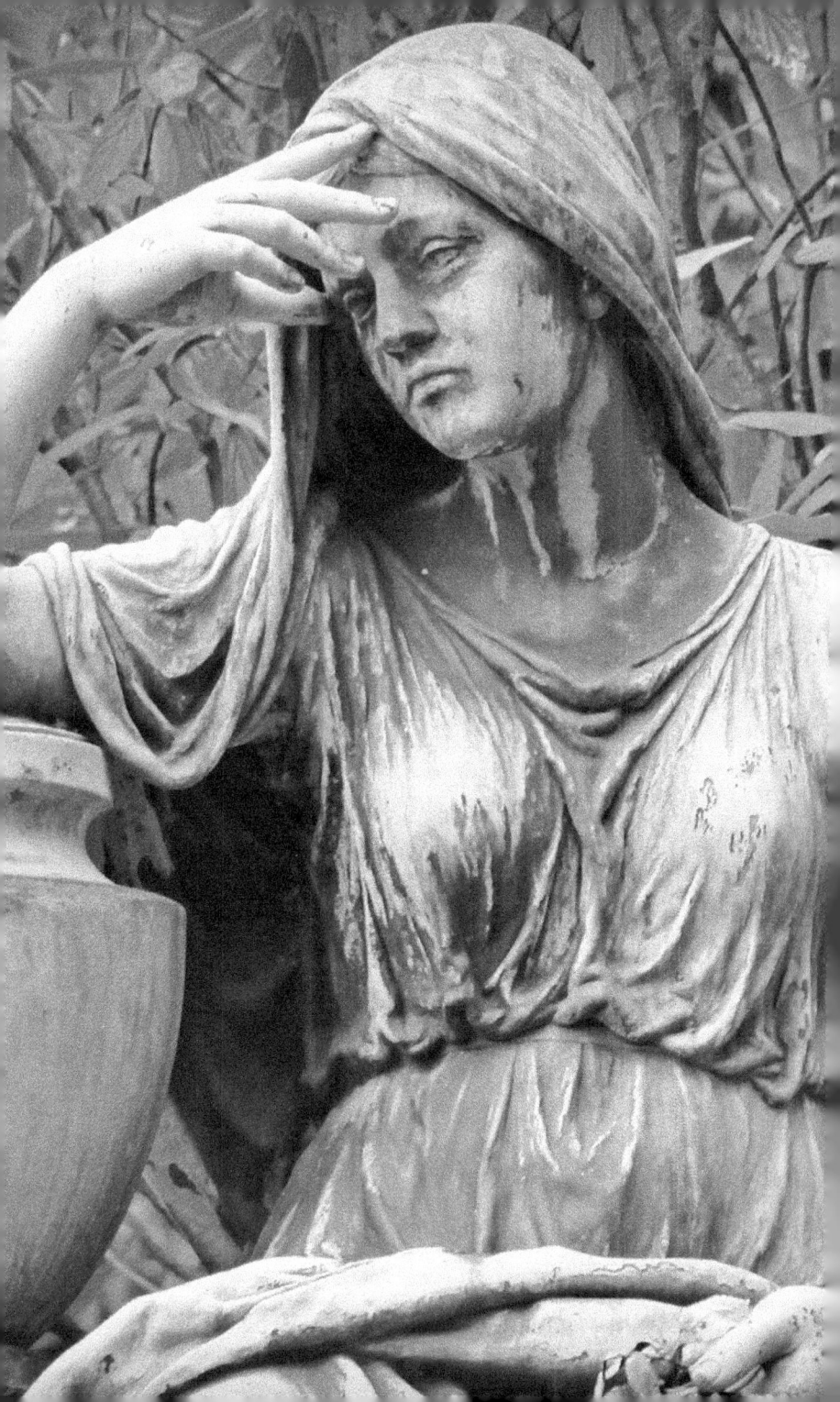

24

Telling My Pain Story

Have I ever told my pain story in full to anyone?

Why not? Was I afraid they wouldn't want to know, or they wouldn't really listen, or understand?

Today, I will find someone to talk to. A friend, a sibling, a therapist. My dog or cat. The tree in the backyard.

I will ask them to listen and not try to make it all better, not try to fix me—just witness me in silence. I will let them know that this is the most helpful and healing thing they can do for me right now.

Today I will tell someone my whole story without holding back for their sake.

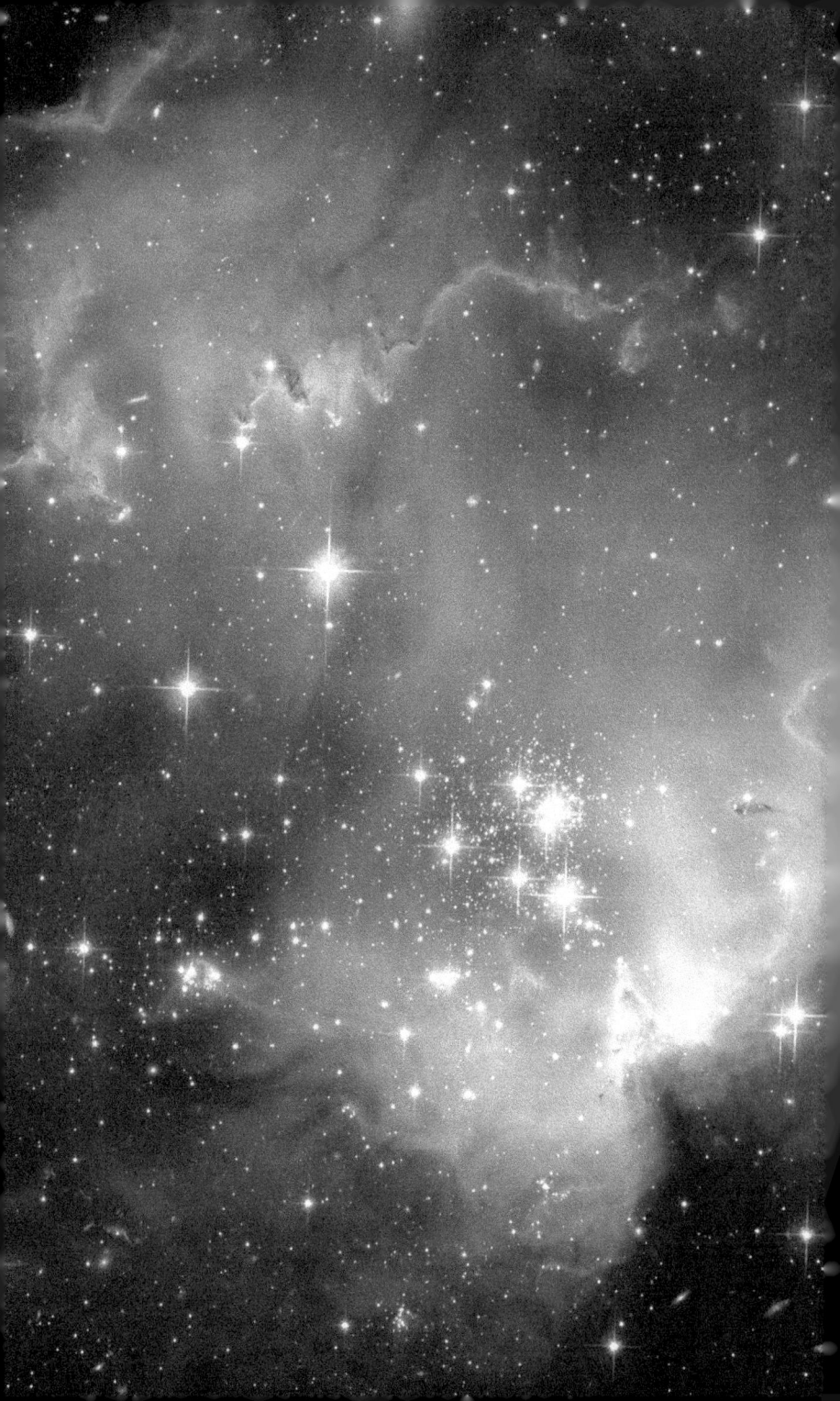

25

I Exist

I am here. I exist.

Pain is here with me, but pain has not erased or
diminished me.

Pain has its own space, and I am in that space
too, with pain, but I am also everywhere pain isn't.

I am larger than this pain, and I exist beyond it
and outside of it too.

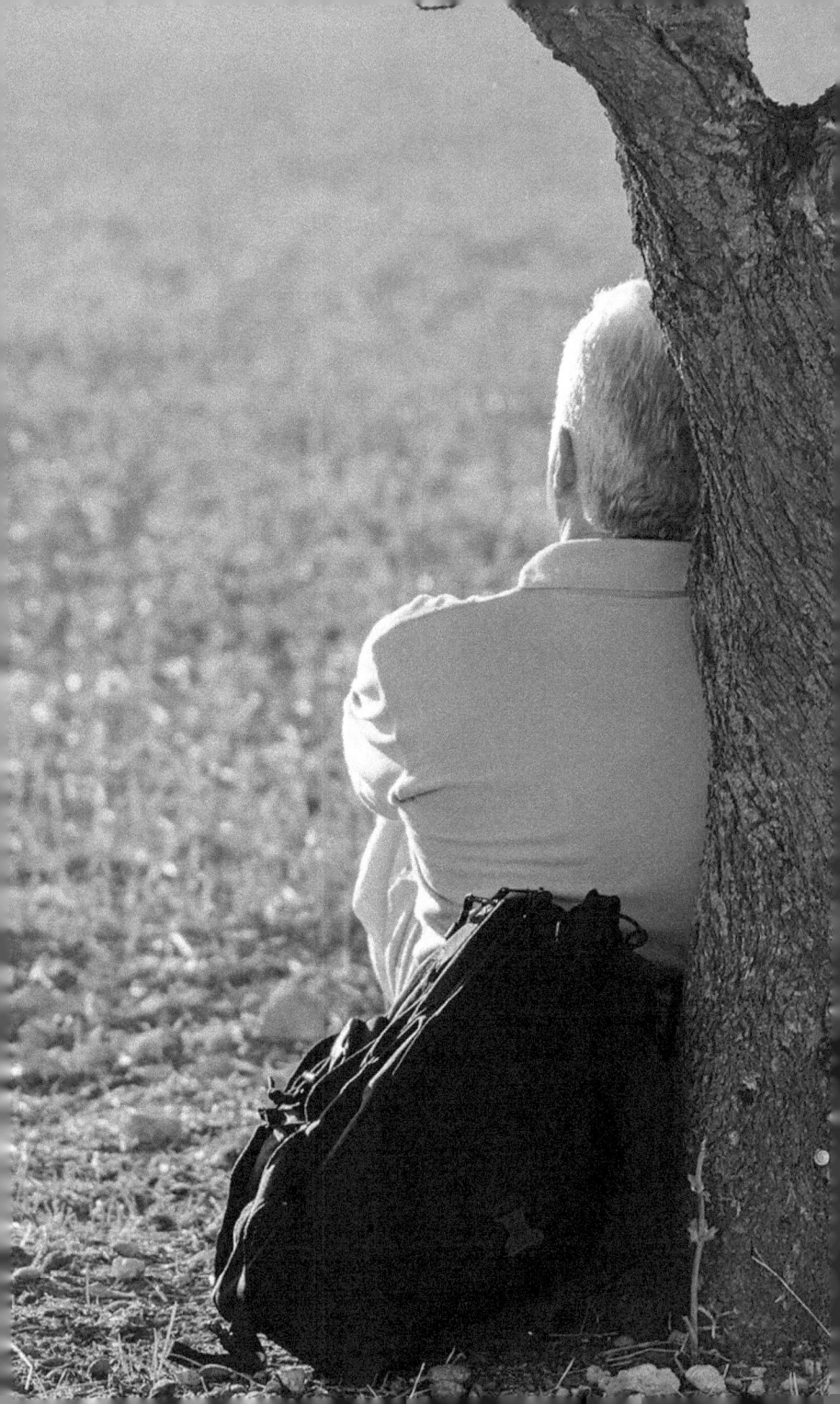

26

Witnessing Myself

Today, I tell my pain story in a different way: I tell it to myself.

I speak earnestly into the mirror and give myself my full attention. Or I say it outside in Nature and listen to the sound of my own voice speaking what's true for me. Or I type into a computer and read my story back out loud or speak it into a recorder and listen to my voice, to my experiences.

Today, I tell my story for the purpose of hearing what is most important to me about it—not for the purpose of judging or making myself wrong, but to give myself my full attention—to be here for myself and to witness my journey in my own words. Words not meant for anyone else's ears.

27
The Bridge

How will I move through these days with pain as my companion, without losing myself totally to its demands?

What can I imagine creating as part of this journey that allows pain the space it needs but also allows me the space to grow as a person?

How can I create a bridge from the person I was, through this time with pain to the person I am becoming?

What does it mean to have lived through this?

How can I best get to know myself now that I have been initiated in this trial by fire?

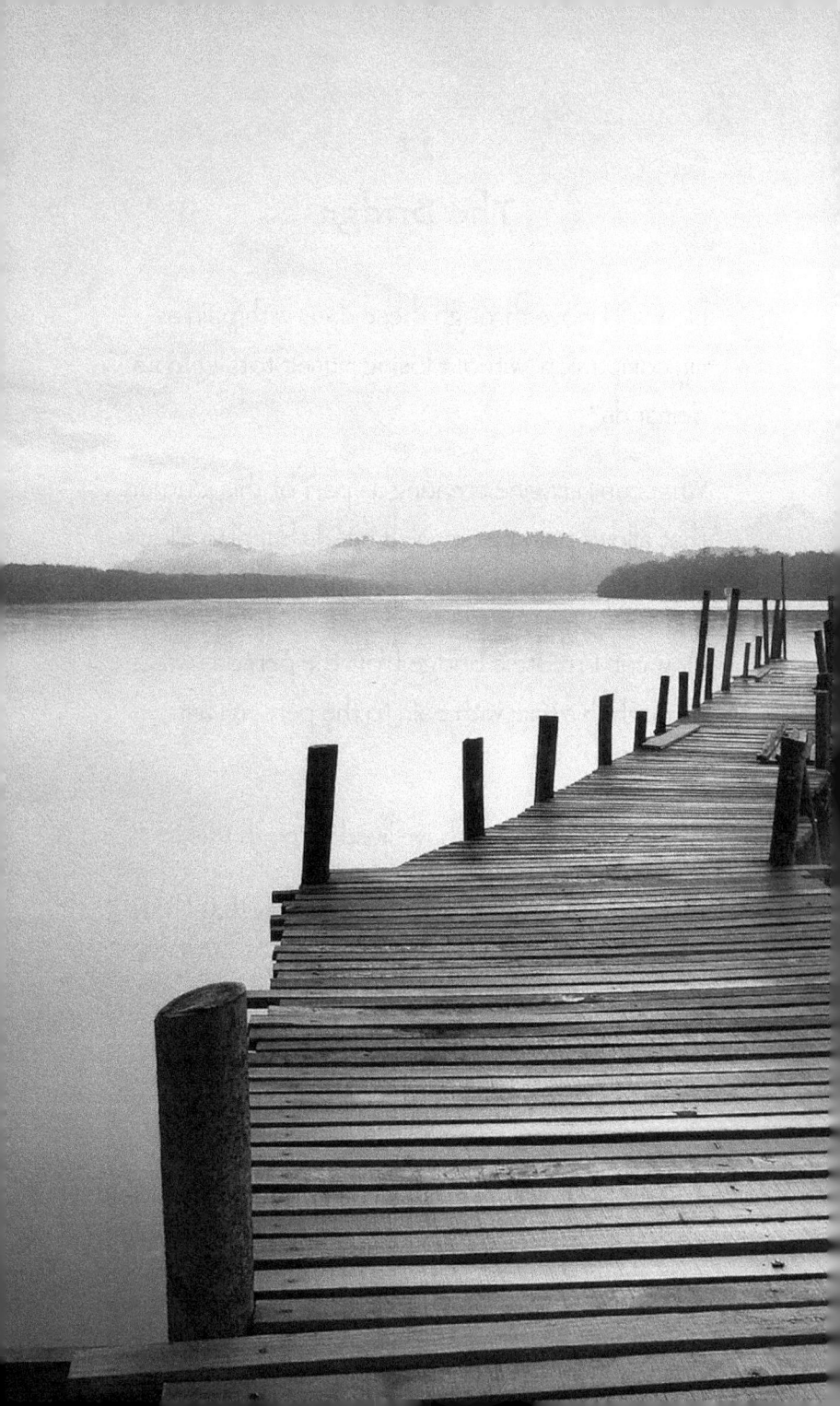

28

Who Am I Now?

Who am I in this pain?

How has my identity shifted? How has the way I think about myself changed?

How has pain affected me, not just in the sense of its restrictions, but in the sense of what I've grown into?

Who will I be when I come out of this? Who do I want to be?

Today, I create a new path for myself, taking into account what I have learned from living with pain.

I choose to think of pain not just as something to overcome, but as a teacher who informs me about what I most value and desire in life.

29

Invisible Good

What good does this pain bring me?

Invisible, silent, unseen, perhaps, but has there been a deepening into wisdom, a molding of the self, a burgeoning of compassion?

What can I do that I never thought of doing before?

What comes up for me to be or to do that would never have occurred to me if I hadn't lived through this time with pain?

How will I use this journey with pain to enhance the rest of my life?

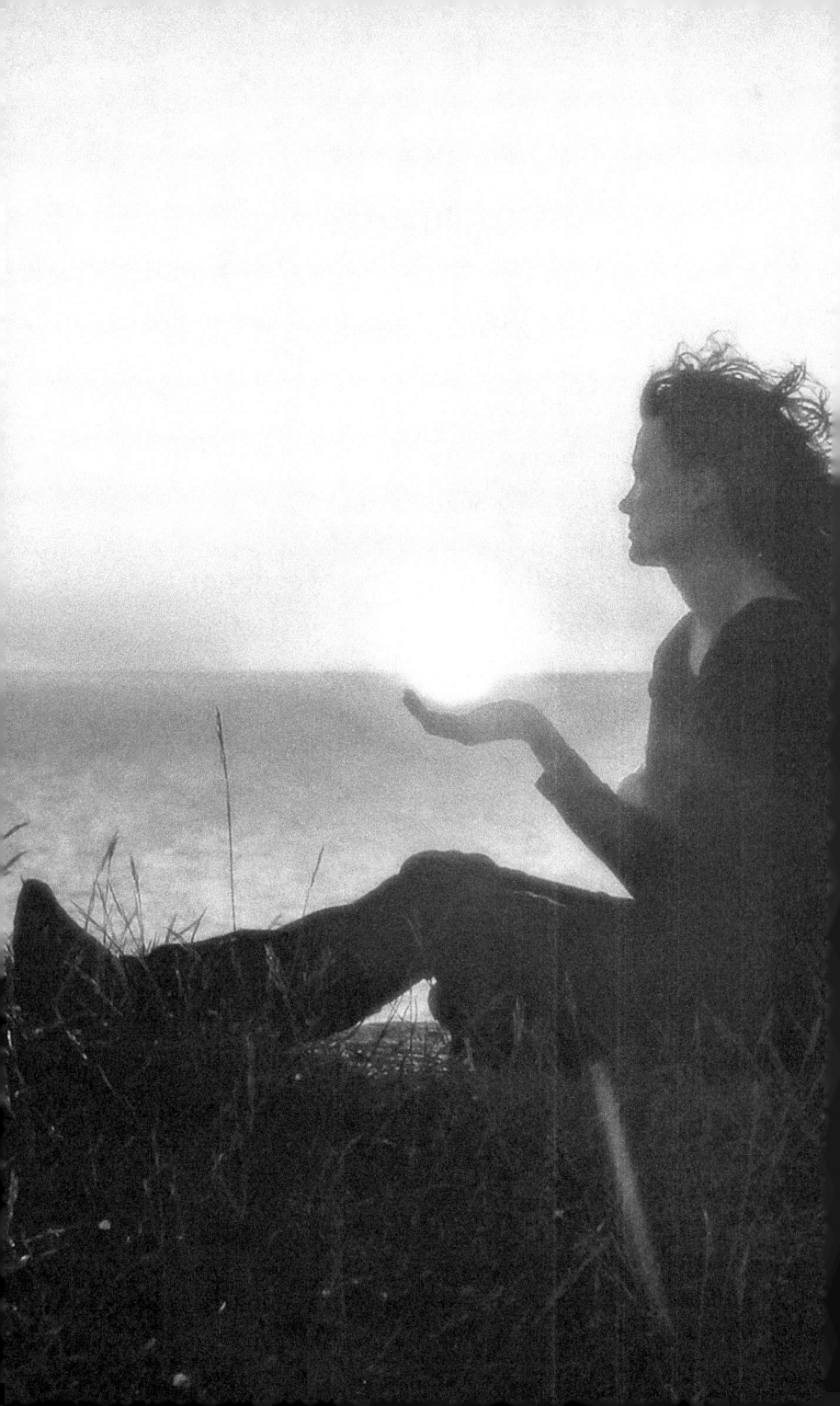

30

What Can I Give?

Pain has brought me difficult and often unrecognized gifts. Some of these I may be able to offer to others who are also in pain.

How can I do that? Do I have insights? Can I create art? Can I write? Can I offer to talk to others just starting out on their pain journey?

Today, the question I ask myself is: What can I give?

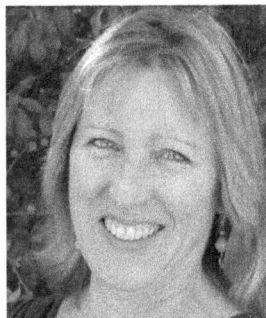

ABOUT THE AUTHOR

A native of Connecticut, Sarah Anne Shockley is a multiple award winning producer and director of educational films, including *Dancing From The Inside Out*, a highly acclaimed documentary on disabled dance. She holds an MBA in International Marketing and has worked in high-tech management, as a corporate trainer, and teaching undergraduate business administration. As the result of a work related injury in the Fall of 2007, Sarah contracted Thoracic Outlet Syndrome (TOS) and has lived with debilitating nerve pain since then. She resides in the San Francisco Bay Area.

Please visit the author's website for free resources including *The Pain Companion Blog* and *The Pain Companion Oasis*: www.thepaincompanioncom.

OTHER BOOKS BY
SARAH ANNE SHOCKLEY

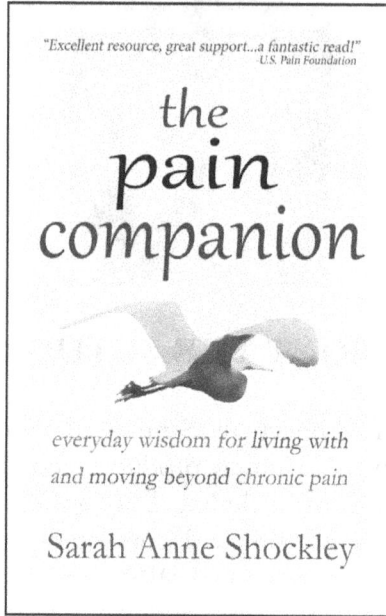

"Excellent resource, great support...a fantastic read!"
-U.S. Pain Foundation

the
pain
companion

everyday wisdom for living with
and moving beyond chronic pain

Sarah Anne Shockley

**The Pain Companion: Everyday Wisdom for
Living With & Moving Beyond Chronic Pain**
198 pages, 14.95 Print, 5.99 Ebook, 9.95 Audio

"Excellent resource. Great support."
-   U. S. Pain Foundation
The Pain Companion is a practical guidebook to:
- create more ease and well being on a daily basis
- relieve the impact that living with pain has on
  well being, self-image and relationships
- alleviate pain's emotional, mental, and physical
  stresses

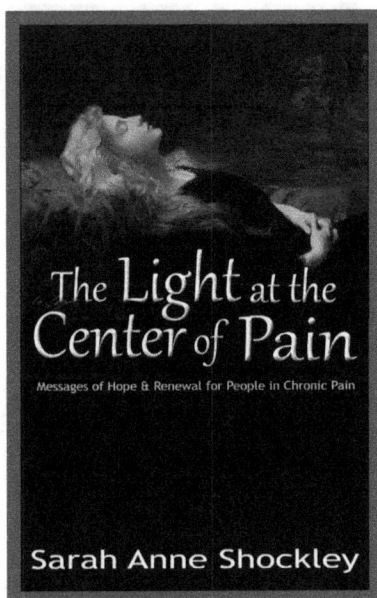

The Light at the Center of Pain: Messages of Hope & Renewal for People in Chronic Pain
138 pages, Print: 12.95, Ebook: 2.99

A collection of essays on living with pain offering compassion, solace, and practical advice taken from first-hand experience: Responding to pain's demands without becoming its emotional hostage, staying in the heart of the self that pain can't touch, and finding a center of peace, even in the midst of pain. Based popular posts from The Pain Companion Blog.

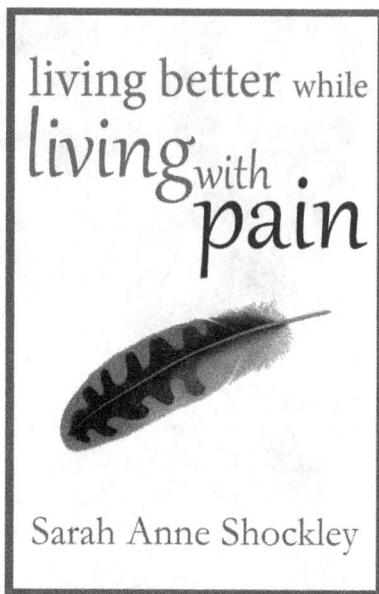

Living Better While Living With Pain
78 pages, 8.98 Print, FREE Ebook, 2.95 Audio

A practical discussion of chronic pain, its differences from short-term pain, and suggestions for approaches to pain management and pain reduction specific to chronic pain. Includes 21 useful tips for creating more ease, comfort, and resiliency.

www.ingramcontent.com/pod-product-compliance
Lightning Source LLC
Chambersburg PA
CBHW071347290326
41933CB00041B/3024